YOUR KNOWLEDGE HAS VALUE

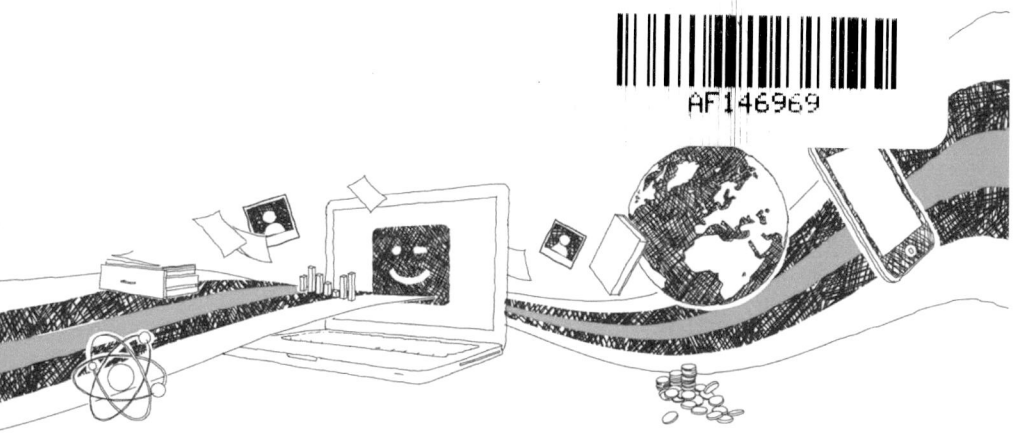

- We will publish your bachelor's and master's thesis, essays and papers

- Your own eBook and book - sold worldwide in all relevant shops

- Earn money with each sale

Upload your text at www.GRIN.com
and publish for free

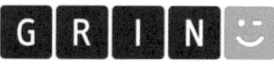

Bibliographic information published by the German National Library:

The German National Library lists this publication in the National Bibliography; detailed bibliographic data are available on the Internet at http://dnb.dnb.de .

This book is copyright material and must not be copied, reproduced, transferred, distributed, leased, licensed or publicly performed or used in any way except as specifically permitted in writing by the publishers, as allowed under the terms and conditions under which it was purchased or as strictly permitted by applicable copyright law. Any unauthorized distribution or use of this text may be a direct infringement of the author s and publisher s rights and those responsible may be liable in law accordingly.

Imprint:

Copyright © 2018 GRIN Verlag
Print and binding: Books on Demand GmbH, Norderstedt Germany
ISBN: 9783668692459

This book at GRIN:

https://www.grin.com/document/423818

Patrick Kimuyu

The Impact of Knowledge, Attitude and Social Norm Changes on Cigarette Smoking Behavior in the United States

GRIN Verlag

GRIN - Your knowledge has value

Since its foundation in 1998, GRIN has specialized in publishing academic texts by students, college teachers and other academics as e-book and printed book. The website www.grin.com is an ideal platform for presenting term papers, final papers, scientific essays, dissertations and specialist books.

Visit us on the internet:

http://www.grin.com/

http://www.facebook.com/grincom

http://www.twitter.com/grin_com

The Impact of Knowledge, Attitude and Social Norm Changes on Cigarette Smoking Behavior in the United States

Name: Patrick Kimuyu

Introduction

In the United States cigarette smoking among youth and young adults is a prominent public health issue/concern. On this note, health compromising consequences has prompted many schools of thought and government agencies to set up programs that support smoking cessation in the United States. Cigarette smoking is a health compromising behavior because current statistics in the country show that it has resulted into approximately 443,000 premature deaths amongst youth and adults (Rodu & Cole, 2009). Therefore, seminar paper discusses the impact of knowledge, attitude, and social norm changes on cigarette smoking behaviors in the United States.

Background Information

Cigarette smoking is one of the leading causes of premature mortality and preventable morbidity in the world. In an annual basis, cigarette smoking has resulted into approximately 443,000 premature deaths, $193 billion in direct healthcare expenditure, and productivity losses in the United States. Despite the fact that the prevalence of cigarette smoking has declined in both adults and young people, the results have stalled over the past five years among the adults. For instance, in 1991 cigarette smoking among youth was 70.1 percent, 70.4 percent in 1999, 58.4 percent in 2003, and 46.3 percent in 2009. Researchers have attributed this decline in cigarette smoking among youth to social norm change approaches such as reduction in advertising, promotions, and tobacco control programs. Moreover, despite the decline in cigarette smoking, other tobacco uses still persist among different groups such as the ethnic minorities and racial groups (Alaska natives and America Indians) (Brian, Shanta & Michael, 2012).

Each day in the US, there are reported cases of 3900 persons aged between 12 and 17 years who smoke their first cigarette? Again, over 1,000 young adults (adolescents) are daily cigarette smokers. The same research further shows that majority of adolescents who smoke are addicted to nicotine at 20. Some of the contributing factors towards the increase in cigarette smoking among the youth are low socio-economic status, high risk sexual behavior, low academic achievements, gay, lesbian, and transgender community. Among the adults, the contributive factors include racial and ethnic differences. Given the increasing prevalence of cigarette smoking among youth and young adults, there is need to identify some of the highly related factors that support smoking cessation that interventions can target in order to have a society free from unnecessary deaths associated with cigarette smoking. Cross sectional survey in the United States show differences in tobacco prevalence among different demographic categories such as age, sex, and race (Brian, Shanta & Michael, 2012). Figure 1, 2 and 3 show this prevalence in the last five years.

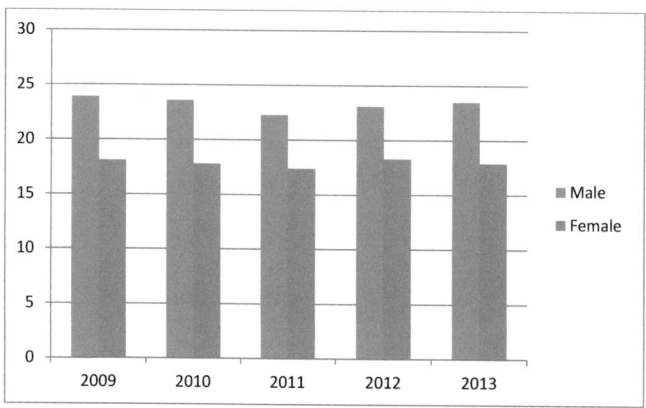

Figure 1: cigarette smoking among persons above 18 years by sex (Palmersheim, 2005).

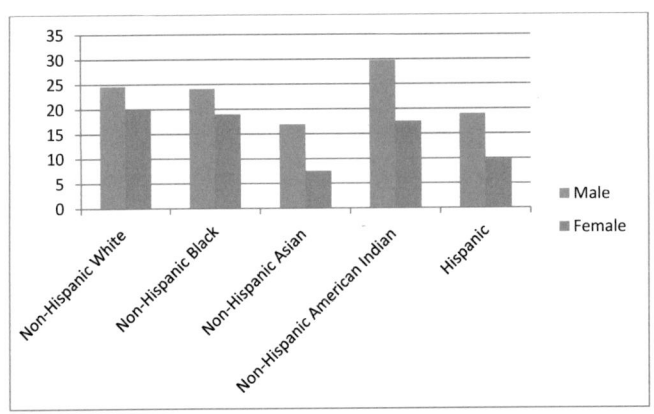

Figure 2 shows cigarette smoking by sex, race, and Hispanic origin (Palmersheim, 2005).

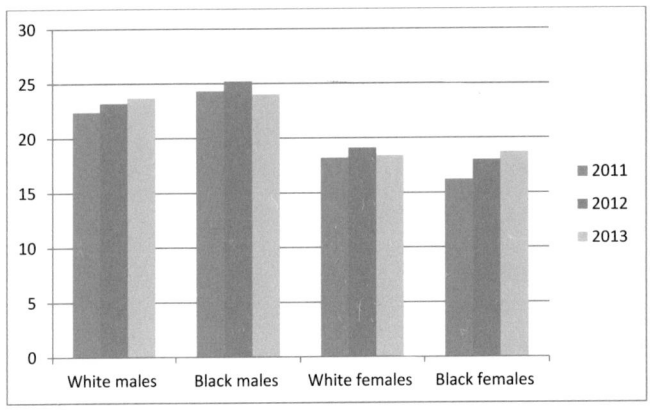

Figure 3 shows cigarette smoking by race and sex (above 18 years) (Palmersheim, 2005).

Research Findings

Knowledge, attitude, and social norm changes are distinct concepts predicting specific behavioral attention and in predicting behavioral change. Some of the social norm changes such as passing tobacco control policies can help in eliminating the hazardous effects of cigarette smoking among youth and young adults (change smoking behaviors). Enacting such policies to stronger anti-smoking norms can help in reducing tobacco smoking based on the fact that smoking related behaviors are not desirable. People can develop attitudes towards the policy at the population level hence represent change in smoking related social norms. For instance, national smoking prevention policies including increasing cigarette excise taxes, banning smoking in public areas, and educating members of the public on the harmful effects of cigarette smoking can support smoking cessation in the United States. These social norm practices will have positive effects on anti-smoking efforts in the United States (Ashley, 2000). The US government has enacted laws intended to restrict smoking in public places, banned all forms of advertising in social media, and also introduced a smoking age of 18 years and above. In the last ten years, the US total score on tobacco control measures has improved considerably due to high health warnings from the government and other programs. Some of the control measures are increased spending on cigarette control, banning advertisements, ban of public smoking places, and health warnings (Zhang, Cowling & Tang, 2010).

The articles have also highlighted that most of the smokers have low levels of health knowledge implying that if health knowledge is increased in the nation, it would reduce smoking rates for instance, adult rates from minority groups. All the six studies have highlighted that both knowledge and attitude are linked with cigarette smoking in the United States although some of the articles have few large surveys investigating the impact of knowledge and attitude towards smoking cigarettes in the United States (Ashley, 2000).

Findings from the articles further shows that cigarette smoking in the United States is highly associated with sex, age, race, education, alcohol drinking, and knowledge about health problems and attitude towards cigarette smoking. For instance, the subjects who had lower attitude score had a higher risk of cigarette smoking in comparison to subjects who had higher attitude score. This implies that attitude in the United States has a significant impact on smoking cessation. The study further shows that subjects who are young with good health think less of health hazards implying that a large number of youths do not pay attention to the available information on health effects of cigarette smoking, and also exposure to secondhand smoke such as smoking at home (Zhang, Cowling & Tang, 2010). There was also a significant relationship between the subjects who had a low level of education (lower knowledge score) and shown a negative attitude towards smoking (lower attitude score) are more likely to engage in smoking practices. In an agreement with the six articles studied, knowledge of the subjects about smoking practices and attitude towards smoking are significantly associated with increased cigarette smoking in the United States. Interestingly, the articles show that the attitude towards smoking is linked with smoking behaviors even when the subjects adjust to potential confounders. A comparison of the three variables (knowledge, attitude, and social norm changes) shows that the attitude towards smoking in the United States was more strongly associated with cigarette smoking among the youth and adults. This implies that those subjects with more negative attitude towards smoking are more likely to be smokers (Ashley, 2000).

The study further shows that the highly educated and older people are less likely to be smokers and higher rates of cigarette smoking are associated with youth and young adults. Interestingly, there was a high level of awareness on the dangers of cigarette smoking whereby 90 percent of the smokers knew that increased cigarette smoking is harmful to their health. One-third of the population investigated in the United States argued that cigarette smoking was the main cause of their illness (health problems). For instance, cancer was mentioned by more than half of the subjects investigated. This implies that most of the subjects had knowledge that cigarette smoking can cause health problems including cancer, but because of their positive attitude towards smoking, they pursued smoking due to different reasons, and the mostly mentioned reasons are social-economic status, dual diagnosis, heavy and long-term smokers, aboriginal people, high risk sexual behavior, and low academic achievements. For the ethnic minorities and racial groups in the United States, large gaps exist in their understanding of the negative effects of cigarette smoking. There are still extremely high levels of misunderstanding on the potential impact of light cigarettes. This is despite the popular support for tobacco control measures in the country (Ma et al, 2005).

Discussion

From the above findings, it can be concluded that knowledge, attitude, and social norm changes have an impact on cigarette smoking behavior in the United States. For instance, knowledge on health problems associated with smoking practices can help in cigarette cessation in the country. It is important to improve the knowledge of all cigarette smokers (youth and adults) on the danger of cigarette smoking so that they can change their attitude and behavior towards cigarette smoking (Ma et al, 2005).

The social norm change paradigm still has an impact on cigarette smoking behavior in the United States. The social norm change indicates that the thoughts, morals, actions, and values of individuals in a community are tempered by their community, and that durable social norm change only happens through changes in the social environment of the local communities. This involves the setting of policies in order to change the broad social norms that surround tobacco use either by directly or indirectly influencing the future tobacco users by creating a legal climate that makes tobacco less desirable and accessible. For instance, NCIs tobacco control Monograph is one of the policies that have been introduced in the country to end cigarette smoking behavior. The program is committed to countering pro-tobacco influences and the secondhand smoke hence quitting smoking behaviors. The government has also introduced an excise tax of US$0.25 and this has had an impact on youth and young adult smokers (adult per capita cigarette consumption reduced). This implies that the social norm change approach has led to meaningful change in cigarette smoking behavior. The two policies in the US, for instance, the NCIs tobacco control Monograph and the secondhand smoke (SHS) have been highly associated with quitting behaviors. The findings show that those smokers with positive attitudes towards the social norm change approaches reported quit attempts. This implies that the social norm changes have played a great role in reducing cigarette smoking in the United States (Hu, Sung & Keeler 2005).

Conclusion

In conclusion, cigarette smoking in the United States is high among youth and young adults because social norm change policies have not been enforced appropriately, knowledge about smoking is minimal, and the attitude towards smoking is high (positive) due to associated factors such as socio-economic status. This implies that knowledge, social norm approaches, and a positive attitude should be enhanced in order to reduce the rate at which cigarette smoking is going at. The findings show that knowledge about the health effects of smoking practices, attitude towards smoking, and social norm policies are associated with cigarettes smoking behavior. These findings are important in the United States because they will be used by public health professionals to develop effective policies and interventions to enhance knowledge on the health problems associated with smoking behaviors hence limit smoking among the youth and young adults in the US. However, future research on the topic is also required to ensure that the

United States rate of cigarette smoking and associated deaths have declined drastically. Based on the above findings on the impact of knowledge, attitude, and social norm changes on cigarette smoking behavior in the United States, future research must determine whether interventions intended to increase support for anti-tobacco policies can play a great role in encouraging current smokers (both youth and young adults) to quit smoking practices or it would discourage non-smokers from their first smoking attempt. This is because theoretically, enhancing public support for anti-tobacco policies will automatically result into enactment of strict anti-tobacco laws whereby when successfully implemented and enforced, they will result into decreased smoking prevalence's in the United States, and across the globe. Again, future research should increase more variables with common agreed measures for smoking behavior and also exposure to secondhand smoke, as well. More research is also required on the short-term and long-term impact of smoking bans on health outcomes on the different groups such as minority groups, disadvantaged, young children, youth, and adults.

References

Ashley, J., Cohen, J., Bull, S., Ferrence, R., Poland, B., Pederson, L., & Gao, J. (2000). Knowledge about tobacco and attitudes toward tobacco control: how different are smokers and nonsmokers? *Can J Public Health, 91*, 376–80.

Brian, K., Shanta, D., & Michael, T. (2012). Current Tobacco Use among Adults in the United States: Findings from the National Adult Tobacco Survey. *American Journal of Public Health*, 1-6.

Hu TW, Sung HY, Keeler TE. (2005). Reducing cigarette consumption in California: Tobacco taxes vs. an anti-smoking media campaign. *Am J Public Health, 85*, 1218e22.

Ma, X., Tan, Y., Fang, Y., Toubbeh, I., & Shive, E. (2005). Knowledge, attitudes and behavior regarding secondhand smoke among Asian Americans. *Prev Med., 41*, 446–53.

Rodu, B., & Cole, P. (2009). Smoking prevalence: a comparison of two American surveys. *Public Health, 123*, 598--601.

Zhang, X., Cowling, D., & Tang, H. (2010). The Impact of Social Norm Change Strategies on smokers Quitting behaviors. *Tobacco Control, 19*(1), 51-55.

YOUR KNOWLEDGE HAS VALUE

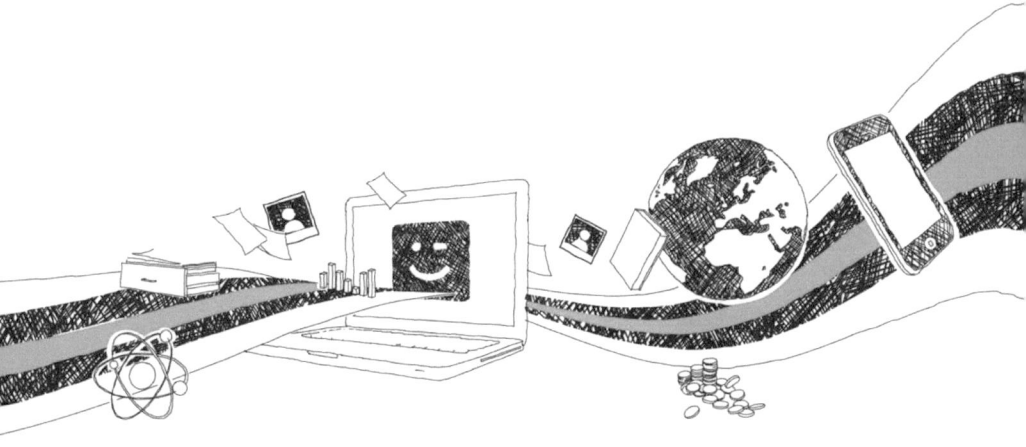

- We will publish your bachelor's and master's thesis, essays and papers

- Your own eBook and book - sold worldwide in all relevant shops

- Earn money with each sale

Upload your text at www.GRIN.com
and publish for free

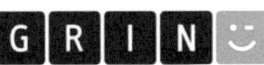